Keep Moving

Creating a Life After Loss

HOLLY ROSE HOLLAND

ISBN: 978-1-7772884-0-2
ISBN: 978-1-7772884-1-9
ISBN: 978-1-7772884-2-6

'Grief is hard to deal with, but Holly's book is like a warm, understanding hug.'

'Holly's personal account of her family's battle with Pancreatic Cancer is brave, inspirational, and offers a comforting guide to those fighting their own war with this terrible disease.'

'We all fear the C word - cancer. When and if it comes, your world turns upside down in an instant. Holly has gently opened her heart through her grief and brought us along her journey.
Through the tears, you feel her compassion and gain her wisdom learned.'
{{{hugs}}}

This book is dedicated to Mike and the health professionals who work with the terminally ill every day. They have two different strengths, and both are equally inspiring. Both have contributed all they have and more.

I hope this will inspire you to support, address what is needed, set yourself free and find a way to improve the world, as they both do.

I also wish to raise awareness of Pancreatic Cancer. It is often undetected until the later stages. We need to find a cure for cancer, and some effective treatments for Pancreatic Cancer.

Contents

Acknowledgements

My husband, Mike Rogoschewsky, lost his fight with Pancreatic Cancer in April 2009. The cancer was difficult to diagnose. It is important to raise awareness about this disease.

I have had the support of Karen McDermott from the very beginning. Without her, this book may not have been written. The trip to Crom Castle in Northern Ireland, along with meeting Shelly Yorgeson, was the beginning of a life change and support from many, including authors from around the world I'd the pleasure of meeting there. The intuitive community has also helped shape a new direction.

Friends and family have awaited this first book for a long time. I appreciate all of you and will not list here as I will be sure to forget someone. In being therapeutic, it has taken a while to complete. Some things I have written about in the book were also true for me in a bigger capacity once I began the writing process. As much as I want to help others, this has been invaluable for me.

The greatest achievement for my husband and myself is our two sons, Christopher and Ryan. My sons are also the reason I could socialize early, as it seemed to be the best method for all of us to continue on. Keeping busy was key to not dwelling on the past and being open to something new. New was so much easier than familiar.

Many of you spent hours with us, getting us through a very difficult time, including family, friends, the hockey and school communities. It is much appreciated, and there are too many of you to name you all.

Thank you to each of you who read this book. I hope you will take something away from here for yourself or someone that might need this. We all have our experiences around grief, death and dying. This contains my family's experience. I hope it will inspire you to Keep Moving.

I also wish to note here that losing a job or loss of the life you once knew because of traumatic situations or a serious illness can also hold a deep type of grief for the entire family. This is rarely acknowledged as much as from death. Both need to be acknowledged and grieved for and are equally important to find ways to Keep Moving.

Foreword

When I moved to Morinville, Alberta, I found myself to be very lonely. Long-distance calls were expensive at that time. It was just the three of us here: Mike, eight-month-old baby Chris, and me.

I watched two women's daily television shows that aligned with my values. These women were my constant and played a huge part in my getting through the lonely years, later the years of illness and lonely years once again.

While Mike was sick, I realized many people have had little experience with illness or terminal illness. Some relatives and friends do not live long enough to even get the information. However, those who do can benefit from some insight. Some things I learned could save people time, money, and help them prepare for what life is about to throw at them.

One of the biggest surprises was when I realized

most people do not have a will. I can't stress the importance of having a will enough. You want your wishes to be carried out and keep expenses to a minimum. Needing to spend time and money to probate a will can make a difficult situation even worse and drag out an already painful process. This book follows our experience.

At the end of this book, I have included pages you can use as future guidelines should you find yourself in a similar position. You'll find prompts and questions for funeral arrangements, a vision board / bucket list, Will preparation, travel considerations, dietary requirements, pharmacists, long-term care and hospice consideration.

About the Author

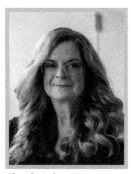

HOLLY ROSE HOLLAND has fifteen years of experience as a spouse, twenty-four years as a parent and eleven years as a survivor, supporting others who are experiencing grief. She will share what she learned and what was

Photo by Delain Witzaney, House of Courtesan

successful. In moving through the grief process, she noticed many people were stuck. They were stuck about death, relationships, employment and often changes in themselves.

Becoming an author is something Holly has always wanted to do. Writing has always brought her a lot of joy.

Holly has also always enjoyed helping people. She has been offering support with essential oils for five years. She travels to share her gifts with others and enjoys nature. Holly travelled to a beautiful castle in Northern Ireland, where she joined other international speakers to network and grow their businesses and authors to learn about the writing and publishing industry, which inspired her even more.

Holly is the owner of Essence Pathways, a wellness business that offers support with a wellness lifestyle and essential oils. She has recently added Intuition to her business.

About this Book

This book was written to pass on the tips I learned that can make a huge difference, both in the comfort of the dying and the help for survivors. It was written at a magical castle in Northern Ireland. The Earl, Countess, butler, maid and cook made us feel most welcome; the staff gave us extraordinary service, and it was a perfect setting to be inspired.

This book outlines the various stages one encounters when an illness arises and is difficult to diagnose. It follows the steps to diagnosis and treatment. Loss of life and finding one's way after are also outlined.

I hope this answers many of your questions and inspires you to Keep Moving.

Holly

Introduction

When my husband of fourteen years died from pancreatic cancer, we continued to be supported by our town in Alberta, Canada. Our support began during Mike's illness. It was overwhelming to receive that kind of support. At one point, I thought to myself; I don't know how I will ever repay these acts of kindness. I knew in my heart I would find a way to give back. As life went on, I found no matter where we went; we had support. Something hard to find after his death was people to listen. In some cases, people perceive the death as the end of the situation. For them, it may be the end, but for the closest survivors it is only the beginning. People do not always relate to or understand the permanency of death. Death will not only affect you at the funeral and then it's over. For the ones closest to the deceased, parts of the death never change.

Time can dull some of them, but those who are close have a permanent situation they deal with every day.

CHAPTER 1

An Ordinary Life

Experience of a Lifetime

In 2007, a movie was filmed at a famous mall, which was a well-known tourist attraction in Edmonton, Alberta, Canada. One night, when Mike came home from work, he mentioned they were still looking for kids for the movie who could skate and swim.

'Sounds like our kids,' he said.

This was not typical of him to even think about. I wondered if he was serious. It was well known there was a famous actor in this movie being filmed in Edmonton. I'd been a huge fan of an actor known for his dancing abilities since another movie of his with dancing in the name. We knew the other stars in the movie were well-known actors too.

The next day, I looked to see about the movie and the application. I realized you needed photos. I clipped one out of a birthday celebration and completed an application for both of our boys. Nothing professional, but what was available at the last minute. I drove to the mall and delivered the applications to Guest Services. They seemed as though they'd been bombarded with applications. I thought that was the last I would hear of it. That evening, I told Mike I'd put their applications in. We received a late call about nine that evening, to the house phone, with the mall's name on the display. I was completely shocked! They wanted the applicants and the rest of our family at the mall at 8 a.m. the next morning. Everyone was to bring a suitcase of winter clothes that had no logos or labels. That was a bit of a scramble because the other three were in bed. As well, the kids did not have a lot of clothes without labels, sayings, or logos on them and we were in the midst of summer. I packed as many clothes as I could find. Mike made himself available to spend the day at the mall. Of course, they would miss school. I was not too concerned about this because they were about to receive some experiential education. It was also rather special to participate in with their dad.

I couldn't go to the mall for the day as I'd already committed to working a volunteer bingo for the minor hockey association. When the bingo was over, I went to the mall to see what they were doing. When the movie personnel spotted me, they invited me to join in as they wanted a family of four. The scene involved walking in an area with the actor known for his dancing movie. That in itself was exciting for me. Filming continued for about another three hours.

We received a call to return about a week later. I picked up the kids from school slightly early, so we could be available for an evening shoot. Part of that shoot involved us sitting on a bench with some of the celebrities. The whole filming experience was a lot of fun. 'Lights, camera, action' and 'Cut, cut, cut' are the words that make me smile with that memory.

All of this took place while we were living an ordinary life. At this time, none of us realized how many times we'd reference this experience in the future.

Giving Back

The opportunity to give back began for us almost immediately. We have all supported people over the years. People have reached out to us in all kinds of ways, and we have been more than willing to help. If you want to check in with me, you are welcome to do so. With the time that has passed and a genuine gratitude for the opportunity to help others start and keep moving, there are no silly questions. I do not get sad when people ask things. I am still moved by emotions and often can't pinpoint what brought the emotion on, but I like to talk things through. It's good for me, and I believe it's good for all of us. My sons and I appreciate our situation and speak daily of Mike. We miss him so much, especially for advice and his humour. We aren't overly sad. We honour his memory.

There is a religious component to our belief. That was a big part of our acceptance. Believing we do see those who have died, in Heaven, was important for us. I consider Mike to be our angel. We have talked about how they are organized up there. Like, 'Are all the Michaels in one room?'

"Having some form of religious or spiritual belief system has been shown to have a positive effect on an individual's ability to cope with the idea of death. Viewing this life as a portion of a greater whole of existence that extends beyond the physical senses can allow for a greater acceptance of the inevitability of death and even hope for what may come after."

DR. NICHOLAS J. NELSON

Change and Communication

I can't emphasize the importance of communicating enough. Not being clear with others can create such bad feelings and stress when not dealt with; it can eat away at you. No matter what is going on in life, communicate. It will take away some of the pain. We do not have to shoulder everything. Some people will say nothing, some will talk, and even more important, some will listen. We missed a lot of years with many people as the kids were growing up. It's one of those things I would change, if I had known how life would play out.

"The things left unsaid sometimes are the hardest to live with. It is important to know that words have power, and even if left unsaid, the mental effect of them can still be felt; however, I believe it is never the wrong time to tell someone how much they mean to you or just how much you appreciate them."

DR. NICHOLAS J. NELSON

Speaking of change, people say you have to just go forward. I disagree with that. I think that is where some people get overwhelmed. You do, however, need to keep moving. In the beginning, I would say at least the first six months, you can feel totally comfortable doing whatever you feel like. If you have to work, that's not a bad thing, as it will get you out of the house and doing something. Probably up to one year, you are in what I call survival mode. You are simply doing the bare bones of what has to be done. After the year, I believe you should keep moving. I always thought it would be forward only, slowly, always forward, feeling a little better.

However, that is not the case. Grief is something that is similar to waves. Sometimes it's going well, and you are three waves or steps ahead. Suddenly you may take one step back. Sometimes, in fact, you end up farther back than you started from. It really depends on how open you are and how much you talk about the situation with yourself and anyone who is supporting you.

"Sometimes it is the smallest steps forward that are the hardest. During the first year after a loss, you may feel like you are just treading water to stay afloat; but it's the techniques and habits you develop during this period that become the personal foundation you will build your new life upon. For this reason, it is important to be purposeful and intentional with creating those habits so you can create the foundation that will best support you."

DR. NICHOLAS J. NELSON

I was surprised with the wave effect and I find that most times you are still going forward or improving, but it is definitely not a steady uphill climb of improvement. It is also not a predictable situation. It will depend if there is a holiday, a birthday, a wedding, what is going on with the weather, your own health and all these things greatly affect how grief affects you. Another thing you need to take into consideration is how much you've been around people who have died and how close you were to them.

What I really want to stress here is not to get down on yourself if you are not meeting your own expectations. Accept where you're at. Go forward as much as possible, but don't worry when you're taking a step back.

I recommend highly you allow yourself to cry and feel the entire situation. You must experience the grief at some time. It is not uncommon for people to stifle crying, especially men. Yes, it is entirely possible to postpone grief, but at some point in your life, to find true peace, you will need to experience the grief and feel it. It is not going away. My style and what I recommend is that you face it head on, right at the beginning. It just sort of flows at the beginning. Later, you will question yourself more. Right at the beginning you are not thinking clearly, and I found it easier to jump right in and deal with things immediately. Often people comment, they do not know what to say after the death. The secret is, there is not a need to actually say anything.

Mike did not want to have a doctor in St. Albert when we originally moved to Alberta. We went back to Regina to his doctor for anything important. When you are stricken with some form of serious illness, you should see your own doctor. Tell them all of your symptoms.

From 2001 onward, Mike visited a local doctor, who he did not see often. When Mike experienced something he could not explain, he did most of his appointments at the walk-in clinic of his Alberta doctor and shared few details about the symptoms. No one possessed a complete list to go on.

From September 2007 to June 2008, Mike received a wide variety of things diagnosed. Diverticulitis, severe back pain and diabetes were the main ones. When diabetes was suggested, Mike got angry. Mike was exhibiting diabetic symptoms, but he was sure it was not diabetes. I believe in most situations and particularly serious ones like this; we know our body.

CHAPTER 2

Last Family Vacation
Out of the Country

Take a family vacation that you have always wanted when a diagnosis comes up. Don't wait, take action right now. In the case of out of country travel, first do your research regarding insurance. You may need to stay within your own country. The prime time to go on these vacations is before any diagnosis. If everyone is healthy, go on a special vacation now.

We went to Disney World. It was honestly such a miserable trip. There were on the way to the airport. Extreme pain won out over communication. The three of us, of course, had no idea what kind of pain Mike was dealing with. In fact, we knew almost nothing about what was going on. Just before we left Canada, I found three liquid Pepto Bismol bottles laying horizontally in the dresser, with little explanation from Mike when questioned, except that he was good to travel. In all reality and honesty, this is something that is rarely talked about. This is one of the many reasons the whole family has a chronic disease, whatever the disease is. The family takes the brunt of the patient's frustration, while they are tiptoeing on eggshells and trying their hardest to meet the family member's every need. Tension is high, and no one knows what to do or say. Many family members of chronically ill patients have expressed their frustration about this to me. Like, the family are not mind readers and they truly are just doing their best, often with little information to go on.

Our trip there involved stops in Minneapolis on the way to Orlando. On the way there, with an unexpected early arrival, we found time to go to a well-known enormous mall in Minneapolis. What a surprise! I did not even know it was there. We got to the Lego store just before we needed to go back to the airport. We took a quick look, but there was no time to buy anything. Time was tight, and I'd already checked in the luggage. We found the Lego store downtown the first day of our visit. It was the best store the kids ever experienced.

I am glad we went to Orlando, since it was our last opportunity to travel out of the country with insurance as a family. I think the kids liked the water park most of all, although there were a lot of good parts. I could not convince anyone to go to a themed water park until the last day. As soon as we got near the water, the kids jumped on tubes and headed down the lazy river. We were slow grabbing tubes for ourselves. They were together way ahead of us, so all was good. They could not leave the park either, thankfully, not without an adult with the correct fingerprint. After Mike and I followed them around a full trip without catching up to them, I got out and waited for them to show up. There was one large rock formation in the middle of one area, which was the only time we could not see clear across the river. They'd obviously been on the other side. It is really a fun place to be, with many water devices getting you wet along the way. In a few minutes, they arrived at the spot where I was waiting, and Mike, shortly after. The kids bought themselves some adventurous time alone.

The kids loved building Lego in their own

room, with their own TV. They spent almost all the time we were at the townhouse in their own room. There were few happy moments and I'm realizing, even as I write this, that I expected the kids to be happier. I mean, they were young, eight and twelve. Why should they be pretending they were happy? An aha moment for me. At one point I said, 'I'm not sure why we didn't just stay home.' I'd no idea how much pain there was or that our lives were about to change forever.

One highlight of the trip was at a theme park that included a safari. We were chosen to receive special passes, which made that park more manageable. They gifted us lanyards that took us to the front of the line for seven rides, as they were celebrating a second round of special celebrations. We went on rides we would not have been able to wait a long time for. Mike found it difficult to stand. We all really enjoyed that day.

I strongly suspect they looked for people who appeared ill. I really can't thank the theme park enough. Without these passes, we truthfully would barely have seen anything. Having the passes, all of us had to keep smiling and embracing the fun.

Besides Orlando itself, we went to Cocoa Beach for a few days. We all splashed and swam in the ocean and enjoyed some time on the beach. This was our favourite time as a family.

We spent a day at a well-known area for astronauts, which was Mike's favourite part of the trip. We toured everything, including the launch pads. The size of everything there is gigantic. We also went on a ride to learn about space travel, which was one of the most fun of the entire trip. I will never forget how you lift off, veer away to one side, then straighten, just as it appears on the news. It was my favourite ride. You definitely want all the change out of your pockets for this one. Change will rain down on anyone below.

The trip home was a disaster. Mike found a deal on seven suitcases and insisted we use several of them on the way home. I believe it was three new ones that we used, but we already owned three. We also had a laptop and my purse. I had four things to manage at the airport, including two large suitcases, the laptop and my purse. Both shoulders and hands were full. I believe Chris had two and Mike and Ryan one each, plus carry-ons. Not exactly sure, but believe me, there was a crazy number of bags and carry-ons. After returning the rental car, I needed to navigate the escalator with the four pieces of luggage. Did I mention the escalator was a single person wide? Yep, and I am terrified of escalators, having caught a heel in one a few years ago. There were no stairs or elevator, so I somehow jumped on and overlapped the suitcases behind me and made it up. My family was way ahead of me.

When we checked in for the flight, the attendant reminded us that we were supposed to be having fun. We were on vacation. This was one of the most stressful days of the whole vacation. I couldn't carry anymore or carry it fast enough. I was in charge of any and every travel document. I don't remember the actual flights home, to be honest, which in all likelihood is a good thing.

CHAPTER 3

Something was Terribly Wrong

We'd some days left on our theme park passes and I called to confirm they were indeed lifetime passes once we returned home. People I knew had not heard of this before, and I was questioning this myself. The answer I got was 'They don't expire, unless you expire'. At that moment, I brushed the comment off as that definitely does not apply to us. I was immersed in getting the family back into routine, always a little hectic. My work consisted of transcribing thesis and medical projects from home. My time was flexible, while my deadlines were set.

We registered the boys for ball hockey in the evening the week following our return from

Orlando. In the first couple of days, Mike was feeling terrible. Another parent took him to the hospital during ball hockey, the first of many trips there. A few friends now realized something was very wrong. Our hockey community support began that day. We would go on to make weekly trips to the walk-in clinic or emergency. Various symptoms flared up, and tests were done.

We went in early June for diabetes training, Mike reluctantly. This was the latest diagnosis. We met the primary care nurse, having no idea she would become one of our top resources and support for both Mike and me. An ultrasound was done with plans for an MRI if something showed. Ironically, someone mentioned to me that day that the waiting list for an MRI was six months. Then I received a phone call for a CT scan that was never mentioned before, and it was to occur in one business day. I questioned that, but no details were given, only preparation instructions.

They gave Mike some results on Friday. They were obviously some form of cancer, but he shared this information only with my sons' soccer coach. There was a two-day soccer tournament on Saturday and Sunday. On Saturday, the coach and Mike were talking by themselves at some point. I'd taken the instructions for Monday but knew nothing about the results. The coach's wife died a few years prior, as a result of cancer. On Sunday, it was raining, so Mike sat in the truck even during lunch. At lunchtime, we sat in the coach's tent and he said stuff to me about being totally honest with the kids right away, as soon as you hear. He'd no idea I didn't know Mike already received a diagnosis. I wasn't welcome at doctor's appointments at this time, so I just tried to go about my business.

On Monday, this was all I thought of. I called my parents while Mike was at work and the kids at school, to update them on his situation, pain and what happened on the weekend. Another thing happened that Saturday. A grandparent from our team said something about illness. I can't exactly remember what it was, but it was like she knew something I didn't. I'd known her for quite some time. I could not help wondering what she knew. It was a really weird time for me because it was like others could see it, already heard it or knew it. I was at our local grocery store and someone there also said something. All were more distant in a relationship from him, and yet they just seemed to know. I am not sure if they saw something or if they just had a feeling.

My parents had their good friends staying with them and all were coming to Edmonton on Wednesday. They tried to cheer me up and brush this information off. I shared the coach's and the grandmother's comments. When my parents and their friends arrived, they all had a look of grave concern that acknowledged they understood now that something serious was wrong. All went for supper except Mike, who went to bed. He was extremely tired and in pain. He was still going to work around his appointments.

On Thursday, the next day, the boys went to my hometown with my parents. Mike went for the results of his CT scan.

CHAPTER 4

Appointments, Prepare, Action

When Mike came home from his doctor's appointment, I was standing out on the lawn, watering. I will always remember how insignificant that was, at a time that was so important. I was probably in denial because I'd already checked a well-known medical clinic symptom checker. It said cancer on seven of nine possibilities. Mike had also checked the same medical clinic and also felt it was cancer. He was diagnosed with stage four pancreatic cancer with two to three months to live. He'd known he had liver cancer since the Friday before the tournament, but they did the CT scan to look for the source. It began in the pancreas. That was the last day Mike went to work.

He stopped to tell my best friend about his diagnosis. She came over as soon as she returned to town. She spent the next ten months with me. We drove to the kids' sports, and she accompanied me at the hospice, and many places in between. We were always talking about it. I always felt the whole situation was something I knew nothing about. She listened and gave me perspective throughout his illness. Her husband was there whenever he was home. His job placed him on the road most of the time. The kids in our families were close, and it felt like we'd blended our families. Another set of friends was also there for us, driving to the hospital, getting him back into bed, repairing, assembling and visiting. There were also many hockey friends, and we spent many fun times with them. I could fill a chapter if I listed them all. I don't want to miss anyone. All of you who touched us mean the world to us.

We told the kids the next day about Mike's cancer, over the telephone, because they weren't due back for a few days. We felt we needed to tell them as soon as we could. They were attending an event on Thursday with my parents when we got the news. We did not say anything about the two to three-month part, hoping and praying for a cure.

When you receive a terminal illness diagnosis, people seem to either act immediately or be paralyzed. We took action with a trip to our lawyer the morning after the diagnosis. Filling out the appropriate paperwork is critical. The rules can vary by country. It seems morbid to be preparing for death, but it is a huge gift to the survivors. You will know and be ready to carry out their wishes. In the case of spouses, it is also simpler, because at least in Canada, you can keep it out of court saving time and money. Your bills still need to be paid. Sometimes joint accounts are frozen as well, although not the norm. You can do simple things like putting money into an account only in your name or making an extra bill payment will buy you time afterward. Some things need time to address, so the sooner the better, for example, land transfers. None of us are here forever, so being prepared is a good thing, regardless. We drew up the same papers for each of us. I believe that was also comforting to Mike. It put us more on a level playing field. We'd drawn up a will when our first child was about eighteen months. Try not to do this just before a vacation, as we did. We were so stressed out making decisions for our child; it made for a tense start to the vacation. Too much thinking about 'What ifs!'

Be aware that appointing guardians can be complicated. This is because the preference is for them to live in the same province here in Canada. The fact is often you don't know someone or do not feel that is the choicest person to possibly leave your children with. As well, you will need to appoint another person to control your finances to avoid a potential conflict of interest.

At no time do I want to need palliative care at all. We don't get to choose that kind of thing, but if possible, I wish to die in my sleep. I would choose a Do Not Resuscitate Order, also known as a DNR in Canada. Definitely seek legal advice in that the rules can vary greatly from country to country. It also depends who is present when the DNR is presented. Some occupations are obligated to resuscitate, unless the person named in the order is present. Few people are totally informed about this. My best advice is to get both legal and medical advice. Check with your local health authority because some occupations are legally bound and obligated to act in a certain way.

Mike was always very clear the day after diagnosis and well before palliative care about not wishing to be resuscitated. We reviewed it again just before he went into palliative care with our doctor. It is always a good thing to be prepared, in the event something happens. After the fact, you are definitely not thinking clearly. In all honesty, everyone should have a will to make everything simple for the survivors. Something unexpected can happen suddenly to anyone.

Prepare

You can never be too prepared. If you should happen to be lucky enough to be alive with your spouse or other close family member, have a serious conversation with them today. Ask them what they want for the future. How do they desire to live their life, in the event they are terminal? Ask them how they would want things done with their affairs. Get all the details now. It is far easier to carry out their wishes than guess what they are. Write down all the information and include or attach a copy to your will. It could seem morbid, but let's face it, we are all going to die sometime. Being prepared and having something written down to follow takes so much pressure off the survivors. I highly recommend it.

I believe things in life really happen to prepare

us. For several years, I did transcribing from home. I worked for a variety of industries; the majority being in the health field. So many of the topics I transcribed prior to Mike's diagnosis were helpful during the illness. They include primary care networks, Netcare, prescribing by pharmacists, diabetic medications, nurse practitioners, childcare performed by grandparents and babies born with serious health issues whose parents kept a blog. I was both informed of what was available and understood how to apply what I'd learned. Transcribing was a steppingstone for me. I always compared it to reading a book. You must absorb all the information to reflect the correct tense and meaning of the words.

In addition, I was a seasoned hospital visitor. If someone in the family was in the hospital, I would visit them almost every day, depending on if other family members were visiting. I spent a good part of nine years with my aunt through her cancer journey, with many hospital visits. Many relatives spent a lot of time in the hospital, including aunts, uncles and grandparents.

I saw a drastic change in the treatment provided, in particular for cancer. When my aunt had cancer, anti-nausea drugs were only given after the patient was ill from chemotherapy. In her case, this was after every treatment! Every time, it occurred within a few minutes of receiving chemo. When my husband was doing treatment, anti-nausea drugs were run before any treatment was given. I would compare this to the way pain medication works. You always want to stay ahead or at par with medication for pain. I was thankful this new proactive mindset was now a necessary part of the treatment plan. There are many other issues to deal with and a good nausea plan removed one from the list.

Options for treatment at the time of his diagnosis included chemotherapy, surgery, radiation, new drugs, acupuncture and combinations of these. The stage of the tumour and where it is located in the pancreas will affect whether surgery is done. This was never an option for Mike. He was stage 4 when diagnosed and the cancer in the liver was the secondary organ. From what I understand, surgery helps to contain the disease within the pancreas. Survival time for patients with pancreatic cancer as of 2019 is three and a half months to twelve years. (www.pancreatica.org) Slightly more men than women contract pancreatic cancer.

Symptoms could be jaundice, stomach or midback pain, loss of appetite, trouble with digestion, unexplained loss of weight, changes in stool, and recent diabetes. (@worldpancreaticcancerday) The cause of Pancreatic Cancer is unknown, but these risk factors may increase the chance of contracting pancreatic cancer: pancreatitis, family history of pancreatic cancer, excess weight, smoking, diabetes, and age. (@worldpancreaticcancerday) Many diseases have the same symptoms, which makes this disease harder to diagnose. The placement of the pancreas in the body also makes it challenging to detect.

Acupuncture can be effective with some people. Mike did not find it particularly helpful, but he went for a few sessions because he felt better knowing he was doing some type of treatment to potentially help himself. The acupuncturist formerly worked at a cancer center and was trained in traditional medicine as well. I think she gave him some peace of mind. We bought some herbs from her that needed to be brewed for a long time and drank as a tea. Smells particularly nauseated Mike. We'd a burner outside as part of our barbeque. This was the perfect place to make the tea. The special tea had an awful smell. I believe our neighbours may have wondered what we were cooking... and if it was legal. Ha-ha! It consisted of many dried plants, but the only thing I recognized was moss.

Diet is another way of supporting cancer and many terminal illnesses. Starving the cancer of sugar, stopping the overgrowth of yeast, has been found to be helpful in some circumstances. Again, being stage 4, we did not explore this. Pain management was always first on the list. We also tried to get Mike to keep his weight or gain some. We would do our best to eat along with him, encouraging him to digest more calories. There were never any food restrictions. He often ate strange things together. One time, Mike requested cinnamon buns and lemonade. These were two that seemed to combat the metal taste he had in his mouth. He was often plagued with thrush in his mouth. The remedy for this was a mouthwash created by an oncologist. It had a very long name and was available from the cancer center pharmacy.

Chronic illnesses often include inflammation. Essential oils could have been used to support that. They are not cures or prevention. Essential oils are not meant for treating or diagnosing, but they can be excellent for support. There are also many oils that can be used to support pain and also oils that have a warming sensation. Mike would have enjoyed those as he was always cold. Some special oil applications may have also supported him during the illness, including emotion and for calming and sleep. It would have been awesome to have had these tools. The gas fireplace we have now would have also been so welcome. Mike tried to have one installed many years before he died. They turned him down because of the position of the gas meter. New ideas allowed us to change our wood-burning fireplace to gas shortly after he died. I so wish he had the opportunity to experience that heat. It is one of the prime features of our house.

Alternative Therapy

The medical doctor from home gave us some advice through my Mom. He said we'd an excellent cancer center right here and did not recommend any trips out of the country chasing any new treatments. This was really helpful because you do feel you should do anything you can.

A word of caution, while you are waiting for an appointment to investigate cancer, stick to traditional well-known methods of support. The biggest one I would include knowing what I have learned is meditation. We checked into an alternative therapist before the cancer center called Mike. Now I have a greater respect for alternative therapies. However, the one they referred us to was challenging. He prayed on people's desperation and fed us some unnecessary information. He discouraged us from getting a biopsy, claiming it would spread the cancer. We felt sick about this. When I slept on it, I realized it had already spread, as the liver was secondary to the pancreas. We struggled for a nasty day before I remembered that. We put this whole experience to the back of our minds. They would book an appointment with an oncologist after a biopsy was complete.

Mike and I wondered if there were other things we could do while we waited for treatment options. We did some research on the internet and found the study Mike participated in, before they offered it to him. In January 2009, another person with pancreatic cancer would speak on television.

Support from Family

My parents were always there to support us whenever Mike called them, which was often. He hoped they would move back to Morinville, but they'd already settled in Lake Country, a lifelong dream. They told him they would come back anytime he wanted.

My dad would find whatever was missing, which seemed to be everything, especially Mike's glasses. Dad rushed around to find it because the house would return to calm once we found the item. Dad would also drive the boys to sports or play with them. 'He was not too bad for his age,' rumour has it. Dad also did any grocery shopping or errands and yard work.

Mom would make the meals for the family. She would ask Mike every day for his desired meals. She made anything he wished for. His only recommendation was, 'It's perfect the way it is.' This was not a time for any changes. We thought this was hilarious. My mom is an excellent cook and caterer, having catered many meals for up to six hundred at a time. Everyone loves her cooking.

Mike's family also visited many times. We appreciated all the visits. Most of his family was in the next province to the east, Saskatchewan, so it was a long drive for them. I know many of them spent all of their vacation time visiting. They have a very close family.

One thing hard to relay to people was that many foods did not agree with him and smells of everything repulsed him. We needed to figure out the best way to provide meals. As well, my mom loves to bake, so it was hard to restrict that, and we all loved her baking. We made the best use of our barbecue. Mike enjoyed barbecuing and would turn one burner on, put the food on the other side, keep the lid shut and cook a beef roast or ribs like that. We implemented cooking of everything on the barbecue. Mom even did the baking out there. You need to add a bit of cooking time and open the lid as little as possible. If your barbecue has a temperature gauge on the outside, it's even better for monitoring a steady temperature. None of us ever baked on a barbecue, but it kept the house cool, and just required a bit of experimenting. It was also better to keep the noise of cooking outside because banging on the pots and pans was annoying for him.

Insurance

Insurance is something you need to spend time on. If you have any insurance, keep it. This includes health, critical illness, private, company and any other insurance you have. Many critical illness insurance policies have a 60-day notification / survival clause. Once you survive the amount of days, they pay the policy out. Children's insurance policies may be paid until the age of twenty-one if the parent who is dying is the owner of their policy. This would involve a survivor clause. Some policies allow you to add insurance without medical evidence. Talk to your insurance company if you wish to do so and add any insurance as soon as possible. Many patients at the cancer center did not have health insurance. If this is the case, you are limited to the amount and type of treatment you can receive. Often, a work / group policy will cover what is needed.

When you start a job, many places give you basic insurance with no questions asked. Always take at least the basic insurance. It costs so little. At some point, if you wish to have more insurance, I recommend going to a different company. In the event of losing your job, it is good to be approved by insurance that is not company specific or needed. It is valuable to have some approved if you ever leave your job. Be sure to transfer any work insurance promptly. The usual time is thirty to sixty days, but some policies pay benefits for survivors for up to twenty-four months. As well, the transfer can take up to six months, so be sure to give yourself all the lead time that is available. This is very important, as coming off a plan usually means no waiting period, as well medical evidence may not be required.

Before you can collect disability insurance in Canada, first apply for government disability. Some of these rules will vary in each country. There may be other rules, and each person will have to do their own research in their country. This applies to many subjects throughout this book.

CHAPTER 5

Negotiating, Treatment, and Coping

Negotiation

Mike was taking a lot of pills, twenty-four was the minimum. I often made a spreadsheet for them because at times, we also received new ones that we were transitioning into his day. I'd never heard of a pill splitter before his illness. Sometimes I even had to quarter for so many days, then halves, then whole; while going off other pills. The spreadsheet was almost the only way. Tetra packs all wrapped up by the pharmacy were not an option, with the dosages changing so frequently. I would get weekly calls from the pharmacy to see if we needed more pills or different amounts or dosages. Tetra packs also would not have been welcomed by Mike as they would have disrupted negotiations.

Every morning, Mike would say to me, 'I am not taking all of those pills.' In response, I would sound and act as surprised as possible. 'Oh, really?' Eventually I would suggest that as he took eight of one kind, perhaps he could miss one of those. This happened every day, for some daily negotiation. That was one thing in this process he was in control of. My best advice is to look for something the ill person can be in charge of. Everything they know has changed. Early in the illness, Mike gave me a much-appreciated refresher course on parking. He did all the driving before, so I was out of practice in parallel parking and used to driving a small car.

Treatment Days

When doing treatment, we took a bag on wheels that included everything we needed for the day, every time we went. They often thought this was our lunch bag, but there were so many items that were needed, including huge amounts of Kleenex, a blood pressure machine, and a large bag of pills. Sometimes I needed to pull it from a distant parking lot, through the snow.

Every time you went to the cancer center, you needed to have blood work done. Next there was a waiting period and then you saw the oncologist, the pharmacist and any other necessary people. Every day, for every treatment, the volunteers who delivered the coffee and cookies visited us. I found most of them were people who had a family member who'd died from cancer who'd been assisted by the cancer center. The volunteers are incredible! They are so friendly and cheerful. They would even dress up for the special occasions. I remember a super cute outfit for Thanksgiving. They were always so uplifting.

For one particular appointment, I remember Mike being very grumpy. He was usually mellow. I'm not sure what was happening at that time. When he went in for the appointment, I went to thank the receptionist for her understanding. I will never forget her response.

'It is totally fine. I actually understand exactly how he feels. I am a childhood cancer survivor and I am grateful to be here to help others.'

We shared a few tears. The cancer center was brimming with kind and considerate people like this.

The first time the tumours shrunk was so

amazing. It gave us hope. There were two treatment timeframes that resulted in the tumours shrinking. This also brought relief from the pain and he could stop the 24-hour pain meds. This turns your life back to normal-ish, after needing medication every four hours. We were both exhausted at this point, having been on this schedule for about three months. We rested up. A few friends and family visited, and these were when Mike felt his greatest, so they were fantastic visits. We did things we'd been putting off. Let this be a lesson, just do things. There is never a perfect time. Around that time, it seemed like we caught up.

Taking Blood

Bloodwork requires some special attention. For many people, depending on their veins and because there is a lot of blood work, you can't know too much for the ideal situation for taking blood.

Drink plenty of water, not coffee.

Use a warm compress. The cancer center owned a towel warming machine.

When you struggle with this, they have excellent people to help. Some people excel, and you want an expert.

CT Scans

Tastes and smells of the CT drink were also particularly bothersome. There may be ways around it.

Flavours like Kool-Aid and Tang were available for the CT drink. One time it was not offered, and we found out it was donated. Mike really needed it, so for every other CT scan we brought our own flavouring and left some for others. Please note that I do not know what the policy is on flavourings at this time, both if they are allowed and if they are provided / donated.

Reality

Look after the day at hand. I would check the calendar the night before and make sure that day was covered and perhaps the second day. It was too overwhelming to do more than that. A lady once asked me at a waiting room, 'What are we going to do later?' I said, 'The same as now. Focus on just the next day. We are going to have too much time to think about that later. I am just in the moment right now.'

One suggestion for the spouse/friend/child of the patient is to sign up for an online course. Pick one you can complete at your leisure, without any time limit. It might seem odd; however, you will spend a lot of time sitting in waiting rooms with your loved one. Much of this time, you will be alone. At one point, less than six months, and keep in mind it was a ten-month-long journey, I'd read all the magazines of my interests that were available. I could have been learning something fun to get me through the hard times and have me prepared for a new career. This is something I wish I'd done. Another way to manage this one is to utilise library magazines, but honestly, why not learn something useful and uplifting? You could have your own mental escape while in the waiting rooms. Perhaps your loved one wants to talk. If they do, I would of course do that. My husband always was a man of few words during his illness. Nothing like his partying days! Ha-ha. He was particularly funny when enjoying some scotch whiskey.

I also wish I'd written more. I kept a blog. I learned about blogs from a family whose baby died. I'd transcribed their story as part of one of the research projects I worked on. This was a project about many families that included transcribing every cry and sigh. This one in particular, updated a blog daily, so they didn't have to repeat the same sad news time and time again. People could be up to date without intruding. Thanks to a friend for setting me up with the blog for Mike. It was really helpful, and I could leave updates easily. Readers could also leave us messages there. It was priceless when he was in hospice, because people could check his status and when to visit.

Managing Small but Important Details

When you initially tell people the news, there is bound to be a lot of crying. Later, you may have to get people to hold themselves together when visiting. An endless river of tears was too depressing and exhausting for Mike. He appreciated you being the same with him as you have always been. He also enjoyed your best stories and jokes.

People who are very sick do not need you to visit for hours at a time. A short visit is all they can take. The edge of the couch became Mike's symbol for when it was time for people to leave. That was my cue. When he sat on the edge, he wanted to go to bed and people to leave as soon as possible. I was the bad guy rushing people out while he sat on the edge. I have to say; I am not sure anyone ever caught on to the signal. The only time he was up for long was when people came to visit. He was usually good for thirty minutes.

After the diagnosis, we rushed to do the things we knew had to be done, followed closely by what needed to be done. We decided upon a fishing trip to Prince Rupert, including the dome car on the train. This meant we would have insurance, keep travel within Canada and do something as a family before Mike began treatment, as recommended by the cancer center.

We took a train trip to Prince Rupert, British Columbia, on the west coast of Canada. There is a route from Edmonton to Jasper to Prince George to Prince Rupert. There are limited days that the trains run and with the upcoming cancer appointment, we drove to Prince George to make the dates work. My parents also met us in Prince George. We booked the dome car, which has glass on the roof. If you have not had this experience, I highly recommend it. It was so picturesque and was almost empty. It was like a private tour. My parents were there to enjoy the trip, a visit with family and they looked after the kids anytime I needed to be with Mike. The dome car includes your meals, served similar to in an airplane, and there is a large sitting room that includes buffet coffee, tea, other drinks and snacks. The views were awesome! We could see everything so closely all around us.

All of us went deep sea fishing. That was one of the most fun things we ever did as a family. We most definitely still had a very grumpy guy with us, but the fishing was great, and we caught many types of salmon and halibut. At one point, we had to find another salmon area because the whales that were entertaining us, chased all the salmon away. We were excited to see the whales on this tour. It was a bonus.

We also went on a tour to see grizzly bears. That tour was for grizzly bears for part of the summer and whale watching for the rest. We were there at a transitional time and were lucky enough to see both. While headed to the grizzly bear 'channel', we saw whales. More picture opportunities! There were approximately nine bears that came around that day. Most are well known to the guides who accompany the tour. The same bears will come back to the area with their young. The tour makes protecting the bears its priority. There is no talking allowed once you enter a certain point in the tour, as the sound echoes and you will scare all the wildlife, including the bears, away. The sound echoes as it is nestled deep in a canyon. They offer tours on boats that have forty to one hundred passengers.

I will add that we were on the one hundred

passenger option which I loved. I am not sure how comfortable I would have felt on the forty-passenger. This is a tour not to be missed. I absolutely loved it. The amount of people registered for the tour determines which boat they use. When I return, I will ensure I am taking the larger one. Just saying! Mom visited with her sister, who lived in Prince Rupert all of her adult life and raised her family there, while we were on that tour.

We also visited family. We shared some awesome meals and visits together. It became the last time many of us saw each other. My mom's sister and my cousin both died before we could visit them again.

Mike's pain was terrible, so I took on pain control immediately upon diagnosis. I was afraid to leave drugs around in case he overdosed, as his mind was not clear. There were so many pills and I hid the ones we were not actively using at that moment, but might need later, especially becoming toxic so many times. Toxic always meant switching to something new, but sometimes we would go back to the same drug later. This is all part of a huge learning curve, especially if you are not of a medical background.

CHAPTER 6

Research to Improve the Life of Others While Helping Himself

A desire to do whatever he could was high on Mike's priority list. He did a research project about drugs as he was untreated and diagnosed at stage four, both requirements of the study. He had a drug already in use for pancreatic cancer and the research drug was from a well-known drug company. The drug already in use contained about three-quarters of a page of potential side effects. The research drug, almost two pages. It was a double-blind study, meaning we would not know until the end of the study if he'd received the real drug. The oncologist is not told until the end of the study either.

Mike was toxic the day he started chemotherapy. In excruciating pain, extremely difficult to get blood from and in a very unwell state, it couldn't have been more difficult. After the first treatment, he shared his opinion on a death from cancer. 'They must have died a terrible death.'

The day after Mike started treatment was a very low day. I told the research nurse he was undecided whether to continue on. She was not pushy. She simply said that was up to him. I told him I was pretty sure he was on the real drug. Both he, and later, his oncologist was intrigued. As I mentioned, we'd a list of all the potential side effects. Mike showed signs of two new side effects since starting the treatment. They were only on the research drug list. The oncologist was amazing, and she was so excited when we told her.

We were heading into the September long weekend and I was not sure he would survive it. The research nurse booked Mike in to spend a day in a ward as an outpatient. This is where you see all the professionals to help you sort out nutrition, medication, oncologist, dietician, pharmacist, counsellor, nurse and a few other modalities. This really helped because they give you a consensus plan. Most people find one says do this, the other one says do that. In this situation, they all collaborate and give you a group plan they all agree upon. This removes a lot of frustration for the patient. It gave Mike a new view of the whole picture.

There are a lot of questions to answer and forms to complete when participating in research. Mike tired of them early. I would ask him the questions, he answered, and I always wrote the answers down. He felt they should use a photocopier. They were looking for variations, patterns and I'm not sure what else. He was exhausted and just wanted to be left alone. We always got the prescription for the study drug from the cancer center pharmacy, the location he received his treatments. They required us to return the bottle from the prior month. I never counted how many pills were actually in the bottle. I think there was some psychology to see if you would take more pills than one per day, if given the opportunity. I don't know why, but I don't believe either of us ever counted the pills and I don't believe the amount in the bottle was always just the amount you needed each month. I think sometimes there were quite a few extras, and some there was just the right amount. It would be interesting to know what the psychology is behind that.

Both Mike and I were very excited, believing he was taking the real drug. The usual me would have counted those pills religiously every time. I have to say I trusted. The usual me was also much more about control. I think in that situation I realized there was so much I could do nothing about.

One thing of note about studies is that it becomes apparent quickly that research staff make things happen. Regular staff resent their ability to pull strings for you. For example, they will try to get your appointments closer because you have two or three more tests to fit in during a day. The treatment days could be very long, up to twelve hours. When it's already hard, they do their best to make it easier.

When the CT scans took place, much more frequently, more blood work was needed afterward. That would be two days at the cancer center, so a third day out was not welcome to check his blood. I put my knowledge about the medical system to use. Many places allowed access to this patient information. All we needed to know was if his bloodwork was identical to the last time. If it was, then he could return to taking his medication for the Diabetic symptoms. I did some detective work to see which place was the most forthcoming with that information. Mike was ecstatic to not make it a third day out.

The research nurse also helped expedite a PICC line (Peripherally inserted central catheter) being installed before the second chemo treatment. Without this, IV treatment of any sort most likely would have not proceeded.

CHAPTER 7

The Unknowns and Managing the Pain

Understandably with all the lights, the actors get very warm. Mike was incredibly hot while he was ill. This was before it was known that Mike or anyone in the movie had Pancreatic Cancer. I can't help wondering if it existed before filming the movie.

After they announced one of the movie actors had pancreatic cancer, a special interview was advertised. Mike and I were very excited to watch. We felt somewhat of a personal connection to him because of the movie. Both Mike and I were sad and deflated. There was a positive from this. Mike understood more about how this was affecting the whole family from another perspective.

The cancer center contained many very helpful programs for assistance. You could participate in group training that addressed most of your questions. I believe that was mandatory. They'd others like the inpatient I mentioned with the group consensus, counselling, and planning.

The day we were never to come back occurred in January 2009 for Mike and was one of the saddest days. Usually you would rush home, but on that final day, you hated to leave. As many people as I've known who have cancer, that subject never came up before. It is devastating and you don't know what to do. One thing Mike dreaded about getting the news not to come back was, 'What do we have to tell people?' We decided nothing. The diagnosis never changed. The treatment 'bought him more time' but the diagnosis remained the same. We would also miss the staff from the cancer center immensely.

Emotion Overload - What Day?

I believe we often forget to mention the emotions that come along with the diagnosis. It is the entire family that has the disease. When people do not express their true symptoms or tough it out without pain medication, the family suffers. They are irritable about the littlest thing, forgetting or completely missing the point their family is hurting too. The family will want to remember a happy person, not the miserable one with cancer or whatever the chronic condition might be.

It is hard to explain to anyone how hard it is to get up every morning and wonder, is this the day he will die? Every morning we would wait for him to make some noise upstairs, so we knew he was alive. I would check on him before the kids went to school if they wanted to say goodbye. He usually was not up, but I was always afraid he would have died before they went in. It was our doctor who told me I would have to let the kids decide if they wanted to see him after he'd died so they could say their goodbyes. I'd been trying to control that because I thought it would be too hard for them. They warned me people need to be taken care of properly after they die, because of how the body changes. I wanted the kids to see him at his best.

This is another reason being in the hospice can be a good thing. One thing that should be noted is that you should discuss final, after death care with the hospice or whoever is caring for your loved one. Although he was at a hospice, and there were two staff that cared for him immediately after his death, they did not use all the proper practises. I don't believe they expected the kids and I to return. A friend warned me they needed certain measures for optimum appearance, and I assumed a professional place would naturally take care of this. This might sound morbid, but definitely something to be aware of. It is human nature to want to remember our loved ones at their prime.

CHAPTER 8

Leading Up to Final Days

When it comes to saying final goodbyes, it is hard for everyone. I will always remember some people's words. Once again, there is no manual. It is so hard to know what to say or do. The hardest person Mike had to say goodbye to was his brother, but all goodbyes were hard. I am sure those who have passed are watching down on all of us. The last visits were heartbreaking to witness. I asked him if he would like me to have his brother come back again. Mike said no because then he would have to say goodbye again and he just couldn't bear it. When you know you are leaving this world very soon, communication can go a long way. Talk to each other. It is just that simple. Talk about the real issues and the real feelings. You, your peace of mind and your family is worth it!

Make a point of agreeing on a signal between yourself and family members. The day may come that one of you cannot communicate. This was another thing I was not prepared for. There will be no warning. Just one day they are not talking and may not speak again. You will be doing a lot of guessing, like I was.

I'd received a call from a cousin of Mike's near the end of his life. He really wanted to talk to him. They were very close. I wish I could have got him to meet us that day. When I took the message to Mike, he was not talking. I know it was so hard for the cousin not to talk to him again. Although that cousin came to the funeral, we never found the opportunity to visit. He did not come to the funeral lunch. One of my regrets is not talking to him after that. I felt I needed to talk to him in person, but that never happened. Another lesson is to take care of those things immediately. No time here on earth is guaranteed. The cousin himself died before we had the chance to speak.

Becoming the Expert

After telling homecare nurses I needed training in getting him out of bed, as I got more experience, Mike decided I was the best person to take care of him. The trouble all along was not that I didn't know what to do, more like how to do it. I was afraid of hurting him or breaking one of his bones. His body was so thin and fragile. As the time wore on, he became skinnier and skinnier. One day I realized how profound it was and was shocked. He was a foot taller, so I had a few physical limitations. I am proud he felt I was so qualified. I have often wondered what alternate occupation suited me. Since my husband's illness, I have definitely figured out I was never meant to do anything in the medical field. I did my very best to support all the things needed, but I was not comfortable with anything around blood or needles.

We found out our friend's baby was planned for April 20th. Mike immediately told the snowbirds (Canadians going south for the winter or somewhere tropical), he would see them in the spring. My parents and I connected eyes, and I thought to myself, okay, so we have somewhat of a time / life expectancy. He was absolutely certain of this. I'd only witnessed such certainty one other time in the past. My Aunt Mary, who died before my first child was born, realized her life expectancy would not allow her to see my baby born. Throughout her nine years of cancer, she always had something she was looking forward to. Her kids' graduations and weddings were some of them. When I announced my pregnancy, she never said she would see the baby or anything to that effect. I knew then that she would not live until the end of January. She died in October. I am a huge believer we are gifted a fair idea how long our life will be.

CHAPTER 9

Hospice out of Touch

If you don't want to die at home, hospice is the leading place to go. The change from managing at home to needing 24-hour care occurs quickly, within maybe a week. It was the fifth toxic to the medication time frame, which makes it so much more complicated. Pain is not in control.

If you have carpet, it's hard to get around with an IV pole. An occupational therapist came in and we ordered a bed and some bars. Get support from professionals for this. They are the experts and have excellent suggestions. Unfortunately, the bed did not arrive before he left for the hospice.

The occupational therapist asked about falling, which never happened before, but it happened that same night. The day Mike moved to the hospice; I rode with him in the ambulance. I'd no idea they were so rough to ride in. You felt every bump! Mike immediately memorized his room number and how to get around at the hospice. Our friend came with us and neither of us remembered the room number, but Mike did. He'd also memorized one of the standardized tests done to assess whether there is a need for hospice.

I was always torn because Mike wanted me to stay overnight at the hospice, while the boys at ages nine and thirteen wanted me to come home. Initially, I stayed three or four nights. I forget exactly how many. The boys asked me one time they were visiting if I would come home with them. Mike agreed, but he looked so sad. I just was so torn. I slept there two more nights before he died. The nurses were pleased when I started sleeping there again because they said he slept better. More guilt feelings! It was loud there and not familiar. I am guessing he also wasn't sure how long he could stay and wanted me near. I was the spokesperson as well, so I left notes when I wasn't there. Once diagnosed, I did the talking 90% of the time for sure, which frustrated some medical people. He was exhausted all the time and did not want to.

We need compassion for terminal care. For the most part, staff at the hospice were very compassionate. Like most occupations these days, I would say that people didn't always use common sense.

The hospice Mike went to did not want to bother with PICC lines. PICC lines need to be flushed once a week. This is beyond what some hospices will do. This was appalling because he already possessed one and it provides the ultimate patient comfort, especially if your veins are collapsing. They initially wouldn't accept him with one. Then they removed it inappropriately. This was really cold and unnecessary. This is an area that needs to be addressed properly by the health care system.

Funeral

I was not in the room when my husband died. I felt so much guilt about that. I honestly believe he planned it that way, but I still felt bad. I'd just been told at the hospice this phase can last for several months. I came back to the room to put something away in the drawer and it was completely silent. I alerted the staff that he did not seem to be breathing. Two nurses arrived and confirmed he was not. It was approximately 6 AM. I drove home to tell the kids and my parents in person myself.

Here is the blog post I entered that day:

'Our special angel, the boys' father and my best friend and husband, has left this life to be in heaven. I have no doubt that one of the happiest people to have him there is his father Joseph, whom I never met. Mike and I met several months after his father's death.

The past week has been a blur. I find when I think back, I'm not sure when things really got worse enough to be super worried... and truthfully, at this point, it really does not matter. When you are with a person so much, it's hard to notice changes... and yet the changes could be fairly dramatic from day-to-day. I haven't meant to leave anyone out of updates. Truthfully, I felt like I was repeating myself and forgetting important details all at the same time. Some days seemed to drag on, yet too many others flew by.

Mike stopped breathing this morning about 6 am. I was at the hospital with him, but I was not in the room at the time. The nurse had just told him I would be right back. When I went into the room, he did not appear to be breathing. She checked and confirmed the worst.

I drove home to tell the boys who were at home, with my Mom and Dad, in person.'

There was relief that Mike's pain was over. I didn't wish pain for him, nor would I for anyone else. Going to sleep peacefully is a death I wish for everyone. In my own grief, I was so overwhelmed I'd completely forgotten people can just never awaken from sleep. Accidental deaths have to be terrible for people, with both the shock and the appearance.

I believe Mike felt his work here on earth was done. Many people took advantage of his generous heart and God-like manner. I am not sure how he forgave some of them. When he realized he was dying, he contacted some. He did not contact all the work-related ones, and several he considered friends at one time, he just didn't bother with. We talked about them and acknowledged, since they had taken major advantage of him, we decided not to contact them. I still wonder how he resolved some awkward situations and what was said. That type of forgiveness would have been a life lesson, but it was none of my business. Some of those situations held us both captive for years. There was immeasurable stress and pain. Unfortunately, we missed many events because of this. Besides the emotional toll, we were suffering financially. I still wonder if we'd repaired the relationships, would Mike still be alive today?

Contact people you wish to know about your illness. Be prepared for others to surface. We all get busy. Sometimes we don't make the time for each other. Times like this remind us to do things in the now, because tomorrow is not a guarantee. People often have regrets after someone dies. You may find the people who show up at the end are some of your greatest and most sincere supporters, while others will completely vanish. Some we'd lost contact with, and time was a factor. We didn't know the research would buy as much time as it did. In hindsight, we probably should have contacted more people. Some feelings were hurt with those not contacted. Please understand and realize we did our best. I used to worry about this, but I can't put energy into it anymore. What is done is done, and we made the decisions with all good intentions.

Unfortunately, in our marriage, high stress and anxiety were the norm. I remember standing at the counter by the phone, stuck there, no idea what to do. Lack of communication can paralyze us. Be kind and be happy for others' success. None of us are perfect. Most people are well-intentioned, and we are all trying to do our best.

The day before the funeral, I suddenly realized I didn't know what to wear. I decided upon all black. The actual funeral is mostly a blur. We ended up with a receiving line before the service. That was not planned. We were actually doing some introductions. I could barely imagine us being part of the funeral. It was almost like I was looking down on it. Afterward, we went to the grave. It still gives me shivers thinking of all of it. I always remember one of our neighbours lining up at the grave with us.

CHAPTER 10

Firsts

Our boys were never school guys, however in the year following diagnosis, it was the prime place for them to escape. I'm so grateful for all the support they received at school. While they were at school, life was still normal. The one class they both struggled with was math. It required so much concentration. In hindsight, early tutoring may have been helpful.

On the actual day of Ryan's birthday, there was a substitute teacher. We could not have been happier to learn it was a favourite teacher of our family. That was such a huge relief. She always reminded me of my mom and was amazing with both boys. I realized when I dropped him off at the classroom, this would be the optimum day he could have under the circumstances.

One of the first things we kept normal after Mike's death was birthday parties. Ryan's 10th birthday was just nine days after his father died. I could not take the joy of a birthday party away. We held a laser tag party. It was just a few hours of happiness and a celebration of making it through the first milestone without his dad. We were all very grateful Mike's death did not occur on Ryan's birthday. That was definitely a worry and on everyone's mind.

Sports were also therapeutic escapes from an uncertain home environment. Friends drove them, as did my parents, and cheered them on. They were also happy to attend professional sports. Someone took them to local professional hockey games, which was another welcome distraction. My dad had his season tickets. That, like many other things, I did my utmost to keep the same. The boys love hockey and the team so much; it would have been too much to lose that as well. Although it is expensive, the team has been so welcome as part of the healing and acceptance process. It was important to keep some aspects of our life prior to Mike's death.

Missing Links

Once Mike was diagnosed, we would stop in frequently to the office. I continued the visits after he died. One reason I went to Mike's office was that I loved his coworkers, and I was genuinely worried about them. I did not want to let go, especially when they came up with endless kindnesses to make our last days the greatest they could be. They visited, called, emailed and were always there, even at the hospice. They really took great care of us. How can I repay those favours? The manager did so much for us in so many ways. They went above and beyond and he was also always there for support. We went to many celebrations and conventions with them over the years. I mourn the loss of the fun times we enjoyed together, and all the laughter. I'm so grateful for the opportunity for Mike to join the company and the doors that opened.

Finishing the School Year

The boys somehow finished the last two months of school. Playing soccer and spending time with friends helped. All of that time is pretty much a blur. I believe I spent most of that time doing paperwork.

In the fall, we needed to somehow get motivated for everything in life. Hockey would drag us all out and through the next school year. For us, the busier the better. Less time to think.

The First Everything

Everyone says things get better once you complete the first thing. Any first for me was kind of like, 'Check. Whew! We made it through another one!' It was a few years before we appreciated the memories.

The first Father's Day gift needed to be made just two months after Mike's death. The elementary teacher planned a gift that could be given in person or left on the grave. That was so appreciated as that was a very hard year.

Truthfully, I think Father's Day and Christmas were the worst holidays to get through. Once the first time passed for each one, there was most definitely a shift for our family. The way we kept going was concentrating on the weekend. Sports, especially hockey season, required a lot of support. We'd 2 to 4 practises and 2 to 4 games most weeks. One kid often needed to get a ride with another family. We went to as many games altogether as we could. Soccer was a bit the same, although the season is much shorter and not nearly as many games and practises weekly. Soccer was easier the second year as we'd amazing coaches for both boys.

We also needed to make sure we were on top of homework. That could occupy a lot of time.

We went on many vacations. When kids are in school, the school times off are always considered high season. I thought it was so important for us. I also learned that once everyone is working, vacation time is difficult to coordinate. The summer was full of travel to many places in Saskatchewan and British Columbia. We visited or stayed places we always said we would go with Mike, but never did. We were not missing those opportunities again.

For our first Christmas without Mike we went on a cruise, just the three of us. When preparing the documentation for the trip from the cruise ship, there were only a few choices. Married and single were the marital status choices. This just came out in passing. I found out that as a widow, I was no longer considered married. This was a kick in the stomach. I certainly did not consider myself single. As you will find noted later, I kept a copy of the death certificate with my lawyer's business card for travelling alone with the boys. I didn't think of a permission letter being needed. Only once did a US border agent question me. I am sure they added a note to our file because I was only required to explain and provide a copy of the death certificate that one time. The death certificate was much to the surprise of both boys, I might add. Up to this point, I'd been able to keep mention of the death certificate away from them.

Our Christmas cruise was to the Caribbean. It was great because we were alone or around people as much as we wanted. There was plenty of food and things to do. We loved it! It was also so beautiful on and off the ship and we had room temperature weather. It was awesome! Our top dessert was Key lime pie from the Florida Keys. Can't wait to go back there again to have another piece. The decorations everywhere were beautiful. They were so huge, proportional to the ship. There was carolling, perfect for me because singing is something I have always loved. Standing around the tree took place on all the stairs with hundreds of people. Entertainment was available every night and day. Everything we did was completely different from any other Christmas. All of us are extreme with comparison, so very different was perfect.

Starting about a month before Christmas,

cards, letters, and flyers arrived, all suggesting a change to the way we celebrated our holidays. We definitely made it that way. My finest advice came from two women from the hockey community who I did not know very well, yet they made me feel like I'd known them forever. Both are no longer with us. I so appreciated one setting me free. I was second-guessing how it played out during Mike's last hours.

She said, 'It's life. You are not supposed to get it right.'

She'd many close people die, and I felt so relieved when she said that.

The other knew exactly the situation. Her husband died, she'd young kids, and he'd also had cancer. She'd experienced many of the same circumstances. She told me to do what was right for us, to expect people to not understand, but look after our well-being first. I have lived by it since. If you are not in the same shoes, it is not easy to understand. Others don't understand the things so important to you and your immediate family. Stick to your needs, others will try to get you to waver, but you know what's right for your family. I was grateful I could thank her shortly before she died because of cancer. She graciously invited me to her home. I'd no idea she was that sick. I just felt I needed to see her, to thank her, and she died a few months later. Listen to those messages to ensure you get those opportunities.

As we set out that first Christmas, to get to the cruise ship port, we were flying from Edmonton, Alberta, Canada to Minneapolis, Minnesota, USA, then Minneapolis to Miami, Florida. While awaiting the first flight, we saw a father playing with about a two-year-old son. It was a pivotal moment for all. I swear I held my breath until we boarded... so many memories came flooding in. We were much delayed in getting to Minneapolis. There were snowstorms across Canada and the US, and de-icing the plane was needed. We ran as fast as we could from one end of the Minneapolis terminal to the other. The boys ran ahead to ensure they held the plane. The captain greeted us, and I told him, 'We now have had our exercise for the day.'

Once we arrived in Miami, we were happy to have a hotel reserved inside the Miami airport. All we needed to do was go up the escalator. That was particularly helpful because there was no transportation to contend with and we would be headed for the cruise ship terminal in a few hours.

The weather cooperated for the remainder of the trip. Well, we did have an extra day at sea, since the waves were too wild to take the tender boats to an island. We were taking seasickness pills. I could partake in the wine and spirits as they left you feeling great and not groggy.

We spent dinner with another family of three. It was great to have other adult and kid conversations. We got some new insight and ideas on what to see and do. They were from Tampa, Florida. We ate with them every evening for a fun recap of the day. They also knew about great beaches around Miami. We were staying for a few days after the cruise, so this was welcome advice. That is the first time I had to ask someone to write down the name of a beach, because I could not make out her words. It was South Beach!

Enough food for kids never seems to be a thing, certainly boys. The endless buffets were awesome for this. A pizza buffet was available every night. I think they had something like forty-two pieces between them. With the buffets, there was something for everyone. Entertainment was the same. Kids couldn't leave the ship without an adult, so both boys were free to roam the ship. I could play the slots or have a drink and the boys could talk to me easily. I was always accessible, yet able to enjoy some adult time. This was because the ship was small and I always sat near the path going through all the areas, convenient for all.

We also enjoyed the entertainment by the serving staff at dinner. Another fun part of the cruise was entertainment every night after dinner, for the whole family. This was new for all of us. All the things that were different were fun.

When the ship was sailing during the day, there was also entertainment in the afternoon. I even played bingo for the first time in years. The reason was the prize was a cruise. Lots of people played who obviously were not regular bingo players. It was another unique experience of holidays. Santa also came to the cruise! All the kids received a gift from him - beach towel/ backpack. A very nice touch and once again, all new.

The cruise also had many day trips you could join. We participated in a glass-bottom boat trip. Unfortunately, we did not see too much in the way of fish. The mission for the boys was getting a starfish. I agreed to buy it because the salesperson insisted it was dry and had no odour. It's hard to tell when you're out at the beach and you have all the open spaces. We did our best to minimize the smell because it was truthfully very fishy in our tiny room on the ship. We did not have a room with a balcony. An inside cabin is the most economical. I would love to sail with a balcony and have coffee and drinks out there. The view would be amazing!

Arriving back to Miami, Florida from the cruise, we had a few days to explore before heading home. We went to South Beach, as recommended by our table companions. It was such a fun place. The beach sand is so wide and also, in many places, hidden. When the cab dropped us off and pointed to a walkway, the beach was nowhere to be seen. At the end of the walk, which was slightly uphill, was a beach like no other. So much sand, so deep and beautiful, it was breathtaking! The view consisted of a deep expanse of sand that vehicles could safely drive across. It made sense this beach was known for being patrolled. We walked a long way down the beach. There are cute cafés, all with unique outdoor patios. A single lane of traffic going each way, with interesting cars driving by, often with loud music. It was beautiful, unique, and it is the perfect place for people watching. When some cars go down the street, you can hear a pin drop. You take in every moment of the vehicle going by. People have filmed several movies and television shows in this area. There are also a lot of unique gift shops.

We went to an amazing basketball game and saw two professional basketball teams, the local team, the visiting team and the cheerleaders. We really enjoyed the game. There is so much happening in the seats. People are very enthusiastic about the game. It is such a fast pace and they are constantly doing promotions. We arrived just as the cheerleaders autograph signing began.

I would totally do that cruise all over again. The only thing the kids did not like was almost no Wi-Fi. The prime place to connect was when we stopped for excursions at the ports.

A cruise is an amazing way to decide on other places to visit. The stay is brief at each port but gives you an idea what the area is like. On average, people gain two pounds a day on a cruise. I found taking in their exercise programs helped.

CHAPTER 11

Look After You Also

Just as with the kids, be sure to look after yourself. Give yourself recovery time, but then find a new passion. Give yourself the gift of doing something entirely different.

What If?

I wondered if I should have done something different as far as lifestyle goes. One reason I embraced essential oils was the focus on a wellness lifestyle. I couldn't help but feel I would get some insight into how to live the healthiest life. I worried about things like what type of cookware to use, what type of cleaners, all that kind of thing, and of course, we have great support from our essential oils. I wondered if it was okay to use the microwave. I wondered if we were supposed to eat that much lettuce. I wondered about his diet. I had so many questions. Was it an environmental cancer? He was over fifty when he was diagnosed. I later learned they test people for environmental cancers who are under forty years of age. I'm uncertain if there was such a statistic when he was diagnosed. At that time, I thought a cancer diagnosis was more like a plan from God, rather than something you could intervene on by making better choices.

A New Normal

One thing I really struggled with after Mike's death was filling my day. The every-four-hour meds, appointments and daily shopping were over. Although I sometimes did not want to talk to people, I made a point of doing so because sooner or later I would have to. Other people avoided me when they saw me. I hoped that would stop soon because it was so awkward and in a small town you will run into each other eventually. There were so many days I got the kids off to school, went home and sat on the couch. Next thing I knew, it was time for them to come home again. I sat and cried all day long. I was in a state of inaction. Weeks went by like this during the day. In the evenings, I was running steady. Both boys were in hockey and that starts the first week of school and goes until March. Sometimes I had one evening off or the odd weekend day, but rarely. Games were 1 to 2 hours away, so we were always on the road. Mondays I did the washing but have no idea what I did the other days.

As much as I am not a fan of routine, keeping one helps you move forward. It can be as simple as having a special drink like coffee every morning. Meet with a friend at least once a week. Have coffee and a chat. Besides this, walk or move somehow every day. It completely changes your perspective. Weather permitting, getting outside in the fresh air is best. I love going out, especially in the sunshine, even on a very cold day. I love getting a clear breath. Find a time every day that you can exercise. For me, that is in the morning before I start my day. It is simpler to just get it done and you feel great all day.

I started work in November. They enabled me to work in a hidden office, so I could cry at my desk. I swear I cried for six months. I was alone, so I didn't have to worry about being seen. Occasionally, I would talk to the supervisor but got the job done in a quiet area. Sometimes people would stop by and they would catch me crying, but that was just part of it. No one questioned that. I was not working with the public. I was grateful for that opportunity.

First anniversary of his death

We spent this day with the three of us. A special song by an Irish band was one of Mike's favourite songs. He loved the part when the doves are released in a live show. We'd watched that video so many times. I tried to find a place to get the doves to release. As I was unsuccessful, I decided to be content with viewing the video. We all took the day in April 2010 off. The three of us spent the day at a Mall Water Park. I told the boys we would not be taking every anniversary day off. This was unique as it was the first. We were in disbelief that a year passed. It flew by and dragged all at the same time. All considered, we enjoyed a great day celebrating Mike's life.

Our friends obtained tickets for that favorite Irish band when they played in Edmonton. The boys and I attended the concert with them and it was an amazing celebration of Mike's life and the boys' first concert. Such an epic one.

Magical Year went over my Head

I want to mention there is a book I found really helpful about the year after someone dies. I have included it on my website hollyroseholland.com. Even though I didn't recognize it, I was doing many of the same things. In other situations, I have known of people acting a certain way, noticing others, but not seeing the same behaviour in themselves. It totally was the same for me. Although I knew consciously Mike died and saw him dead with my own eyes, I still visited his office frequently. I finally realized over a year later that besides checking up on coworkers, I went there to find him. It's very hard to explain. It's like your subconscious is taking you to a location just in case they happen to be there.

There seemed to be no end of firsts. That is one thing that always strikes me. They can come so many years later. Weddings are the one event I am still working on not feeling so alone. I have attended four beautiful weddings since Mike's death. They have become easier as the years passed. The first one was seven years later. You have to think of yourself because things will bring back memories. Your most difficult first may be challenging to put into words. Attending weddings has always been a favourite of mine, being a romantic at heart, and I know I will come to really enjoy them again.

CHAPTER 12

Living Life

When it comes to enjoyment, especially for holidays like Christmas, your loved one does not want you to be sad. Have fun for you and your enjoyment. You are supposed to. Do not feel guilty about this. You deserve to be happy. We are meant to go on with our lives.

I remember feeling so guilty early on about having fun without Mike. I'd asked him, before he died, if he would like all of us to go on with our lives. He said yes, but I still felt guilt. I am confident it's natural to feel that way. I rationalize most things I do. I did all I could while he was alive, and I'd his approval to keep living.

I finally went out with friends over a year later,

fourteen months to be exact. It was a drinking and dancing event. I've always loved dancing. It was the first of many bar nights, dances and trips. After about three years, I focused more on travel. We took many family trips.

The three of us went to Hawaii for the second Christmas. It was also a lot of fun! Since that time, we generally spend time with some family members, depending on work schedules.

School Travel

School trips were another vehicle of inspiration. Both kids experienced the benefit from amazing teachers and parents on various trips that would continue long after the trips ended. Some impacts were tremendous in the community. In respect for their occupations and sensitivity to small towns, your identity will remain anonymous. All I can say is thank you from our family. You contributed so much and thank you is so little to say for such a huge contribution to the lives of my kids.

How to Remember

People vary so much on how to remember their loved ones. Some wear the ashes in jewellery. Some people make pillows out of their loved ones' clothes. Others order extra corners for the casket and keep those. There are also tree ornaments. I kept a few special clothes, but never did any of the above. I received some of these as gifts. An important capture of memory was the PowerPoint we played after the funeral. I don't have that as it was on my friend's laptop. I forgot to give her my password for her to finish the night before the funeral. I was thankful she finished it on her own computer. Someone stole it from the car shortly after the funeral. I worked on the PowerPoint as much as I could at the hospice, while he slept. If he wasn't talking, and also at night, I would work on it. He was sleeping many more hours than I was. I struggled to sleep once the world got quiet. Oh, how I could have benefited from the essential oils I now use daily.

I have become more into photos every year. I love them and appreciate them so much. At the time they don't seem as valuable for many, but everyone loves them after. On reflection, I realize life was truly passing me by, and I was missing some of the little things. I try to capture their photo and acknowledge more of them now.

Finding your Passion

One year at summer camp, one son found his passion. After spending the week, I returned to pick him up and attend the awards. He loved the camp. When I had dropped him off, I could not imagine this place would have a huge impact on our life. They were all enthused. There was a raise of hands for those who received overall marks of above 70, then 75, over 80, over 85, over 90 and over 95. He was still there. Wow, with everyone! He had totally found his passion, mentors, and was inspired to believe in himself. He realized he could do anything he worked hard at. We have volunteered with the organization every year since. It was such an inspiring camp.

Both boys turned driving age since Mike's death. That is the hardest thing I have ever supported them in. It was much harder than getting them through graduation. I thought taking them skating was hard! Skating is hard on the back, while driving is hard on everything. I had to sit on my hands most of the time as I did not have my own set of controls. Both took driver training, thank heavens, but I still had to practice with them. That is not something I would like to repeat. It was so stressful. I highly recommend a professional for

Driver training. Living on a farm or large acreage would have been an awesome alternative. I learned to drive on roads flat with the field around, which builds the confidence of all involved.

Raised by the Community

The community raised my kids and I could not be more grateful. The hockey community supported us during the illness and after. This kindness included meals, gift cards, and rides. Some people wore Morinville jerseys at the funeral service and so much more. Our local Junior Hockey Team helped both boys by making them stick boys for the first season after his death. Local businesses provided job opportunities, apprenticeship training, and a training/work program.

People from all areas of life have been incredibly supportive and for that I am beyond grateful. I am figuring out how I can help the most people, especially those needing safety.

CHAPTER 13

Renovations

Several months after Mike's death, we started renovations. We needed to get some things done. We couldn't do any while he was alive, and now some items were a necessity. Things like the furnace, for example. Although many things in the house were overdue for updating and necessary, making changes was also therapeutic. Again, not having everything the same is very important. Fencing needed work. One of our neighbours did most of it with two of his friends. Many years later, the other neighbour did the other side. I was grateful for both.

As we started doing the necessities, other things came up. I always wondered where to start and no matter how hard you try, there is usually something you wish you'd done in a different order. One thing tends to lead to another. Anyone who has renovated knows all about the ongoing saga. I realized it was important to add this in. It was both rewarding and stressful, but also a major project I could focus on.

I was thinking about why it is harder for some to move on. The age of my children forced me to do some things I may have put off had they been older. Having a major project to complete forced me into action. It dragged on long enough as it was, and we were all sick of having everything torn up or messy—even the boys! This is important. The reason for needing a project is I have realized in working with others and their grief is that although it makes life incredibly busy at times, a project will have you focused to achieve an end result. Renovating was tiring and inconvenient but was also a huge gift. It occupied my thoughts. You have to keep going to finish and get the results you are looking forward to. I tend to have a lot of projects going at the same time. I don't like to sit around or waste time. I did much of the work myself. I learned so much. I would totally do a lot myself all over again. I felt like I'd accomplished something. We really enjoy the changes.

There were a few things I needed to get people to help me with. One of the first was carrying drywall. As soon as I arrived home with a load, it began to rain. I managed to get it covered, as we did not have a Tonneau cover yet. I had not been aware of drywall sheets being sold in pairs—too heavy for me. A good friend helped me get them inside.

CHAPTER 14

Reality Check

Face the reality that life will never be the same. Rather than dwell on what is not, lean into something new. If you were like me and many of us, you compare. Last year I did this, and they will never be here to do it again. No, they won't! That was their last time. Instead of dwelling on it, start something new. Friday night was our hardest, but slowly we have all developed new things we do on Fridays. For me, that has evolved to doing nothing on Fridays. I am okay with that. Sometimes I will participate in things, but often I will just stay home, without feeling obligated to do anything. This has changed in the ten years. Be aware we have to be continuously changing and evolving.

It's all about life!

Believe in yourself and know you are meant to go on with life and you can be happy. We don't forget about loved ones. We honour them with permission for ourselves to live. I spend a lot more time creating memories with people. When I have the opportunity to visit them, I do that. I realize more that every day is something to be celebrated.

If you were affected by a job loss, that can be so devastating. As people we take on the responsibility for it happening. Many of the job losses in my world made absolutely no sense. One situation involved the best worker in the organization being terminated! With a job termination, do not give the reason much regard. Often you have no responsibility in the decision. Simply move on knowing this is a loss to the company. You will be missed.

If you did not have the opportunity to say goodbye to your loved one, I have two suggestions. This can also be good for moving past any regrets you have. Talk to those who have passed out loud or write a letter to them. Say whatever is on your mind. They will get the message. Who knows, maybe this is the way they wished to receive it. It is a difficult conversation to have while people are dying.

If you did not have the opportunity to say goodbye to coworkers, it can leave people quite unfinished and be difficult to move on. If someone does attempt to connect with you, that may be helpful. But if they do not, remember, it is their loss.

Excellent communication was critical to keep the boys on point with school. Staff were amazing 99% of the time for stuff that came up. At one time, school was going so rough, even gym class was not going well. I kept the communication open, relating that gym class and lunch were the best parts of the day and the only times he looked forward to. 'Please figure out a way to have a fun class.'

I could never say enough about how valuable tutoring was. The expense was huge, both in terms of money and time. What really mattered was both could graduate, using the resources we could access. Amazing staff, grade advisor with excellent solutions, schoolwork program with top-notch advisor, tutoring, summer school, online textbooks were some resources that made for successful school years. We used both a private and company tutor for different subjects and times of the year.

Both were so dedicated and exceptional in their efforts to assist in success. I would be happy to recommend both.

Another factor also always in play at school was the ramifications of inclusive education. Larger classes, split grades, and inclusive classrooms are not always welcome. Summer school can be a huge gift. Something we should keep in mind is that none of us choose our abilities or lack of them. We are all here doing our best. The person who needs the extra help is not trying to disrupt your day as a parent or teacher. They want to be the same as everyone else. It is no fault of theirs they did not receive the same gifts.

While there were a few roadblocks, the school experience as a whole was amazing. Many thanks go out to Notre Dame Elementary School, Georges H Primeau Middle School and Morinville Community High School. Both sons graduated with an appreciation for all the staff who assisted them, both teachers and support staff. The staff thought of all kinds of incentives, told interesting stories, were excellent mentors, shared their grief experiences and enjoyed their time inspiring the kids. Teachers also came up with excellent fit career options, volunteered their time and made up programming to fill the obvious gaps in education. Thank you does not begin to say what we would like to express as a family. We all recognize what a gift this education truly was, and it will continue to impact our life as the future unfolds.

My Own Personal Development

I have participated in so much personal development. I found the essential oils after being sick for eight months with no resolution. Out of desperation, I tried them because I had nothing else to try, and nothing to lose. Six months later I was rid of the cough and congestion and out of oils. Never did I plan to sell anything. The great part is that the oils really sell themselves. I am happy to share them and suggest potential solutions. It can take some time to figure out, but there is an oil that can support. Once I realized they potentially could have helped support a friend with cancer she had died, I'd never shared any oils with her. I felt so guilty and obligated to share. I dreamt about the oils every night until I decided to share them. Who was I to keep this information away from others?

I was always the person who avoided public speaking, so this has been a huge learning curve, but definitely a good thing for me. I have struggled with blocks. If life is easy, it won't address your hopes and dreams. I really encourage you to make a plan, including a vision board with everything written down, and prepare to achieve your dreams. You really can do anything you focus on. As a lover of the ocean and travel, I work it into every opportunity to learn and grow. The world is out there waiting!

Besides the benefits of moving your body, it is in our best interest to be grounded. One easy way to ground yourself is to spend some time in nature. Go outside and get as close to the ground as you can. Walking on the grass or soil with bare feet is really good for us. Gardening is an amazing way to ground yourself. As it turns out, there are many reasons I like gardening. Some of them I learned only in the past year.

This past year has been a transformational one for me. Writing has been very therapeutic, bringing out emotions I didn't realize were stifled. I am so grateful for the opportunity to unload onto the page. I have also worked on my intuition. As the cellular changes continued, I finished my year of Gratitude and began the next year and decade with Intention.

I am grateful to have found a writers community in the past year. It is amazing to know they totally understand where you are coming from. They share their knowledge generously. When I found the community, I felt as if I had come home.

Gratitude has really helped me. We checked things off Mike's bucket list. When we wanted to do something, we just did. We didn't know how much time we had left. I know we'd previously not gone to events or places because we did not have a lot of time to take in the entire location or event. Do not get bogged down with finishing. The important thing here is to start.

I am incredibly blessed to have two awesome sons. Mike's death was a huge blow to both. For one son, he went everywhere with his dad. For the other, he missed spending time with him. All of us miss Mike more than we can express, but we know he wants the finest of life for all of us.

I discovered another reason I love calligraphy so much. It is because of the flow of energy. I learned this as part of a Qi Gong class I took. Entering on the computer or dictation is faster, but it does not always have the same flow for me. Calligraphy is decorative and beautiful.

Editing this has taken what seems literally like forever. I feel there is some real psychology here. It was so hard to really get into it. I think partly I am viewing its publishing as a learning experience. It is thought-provoking and very exciting, all at the same time. It's all kind of 'pinch me, what's next?' I have many writing projects ahead of me to finish and start but *sigh*, Deep Breath and Smile! I am feeling so grateful to have this opportunity.

I was lucky because my kids were young. I needed to be the one to get them to school and sports. The boys were not so lucky being young and having a short time with their dad.

CHAPTER 15

Success and the Little Things

'How long are we going to live?' Let's be honest, this movie is playing on the mind of all involved. Again, since only the guy upstairs knows how long that is, I was looking for an answer. My best answer was 'My great grandma lived to just short of 100 and that's what I'm shooting for.' This question came up so many times, always at bedtime. This is another one of those many times when you didn't have the answer and could not fix it. I was as reassuring as possible, while being aware not to over promise.

Kindness

During Spring Break, my parents took the boys to British Columbia to their home. I was happy they were away for a break, all four of them. In some ways it was easier for me because we were well into a month of every four-hour medications once again. Once he fell, I needed to make sure someone else was in the house if I needed to go out or if I wanted to take a shower. I also sat on the couch below his room so I could hear him without watching. Many offered to come over, which I was so thankful for. He still requested shopping for me to do, generally every day. A good friend even shopped for my Easter candy that year. I was so grateful. She was going to get hers and offered. I took her up on that. I remember that every year. She and another friend also worked our volunteering hockey concession shifts for us that winter. That was so appreciated.

The teacher who changed Ryan's path offered a visit for the boys to her farm. I wish I'd taken her up on it. They would have loved it. I just couldn't figure out how to get them there. I'm sure they could have caught a ride home with her, but at the time I did not even think of that. Anyway, hindsight gives you all kinds of answers. Her offer, like so many others, was beyond kind. We appreciated all the offers; some we just didn't think of ways to make them work.

Food was always being delivered from the community. At times, I did not take people up on meals because it was hard to feed Mike. So many things upset him. Stomach trouble is a huge part of pancreatic cancer, and, of course, the aromas. Those could change daily, and it was hard to have room to store the food. Mike wanted a new fridge. We purchased one, which he was thrilled with. The small things like that end up being the big things. He made sure we were well set up going forward.

At the funeral, many people offered help. They were so kind, and I was very overwhelmed. I asked at times for things, but thankfully there were no huge situations. I told myself I would try not to ask. It was important to me, not to be needy. People definitely helped. Directions were one of those things I asked for. I was used to driving to half of the hockey arenas, while Mike drove to the other half. I was used to Mike keeping score, as he really enjoyed that and all the action with the penalty box. When he was no longer there, I did a bit of scorekeeping, but mostly I played the music or worked in the concession for the boys' teams. I contributed in the areas I was best at, as Mike did.

About a week after the funeral, I thought about my rings. Was I supposed to keep wearing them and for how long? There it is again. No one asked much about them, but it was another major thing I was unsure about. My fingers were sore every morning. After about six months, I stopped wearing my engagement and wedding ring. My fingers were just too sore. Someone pulled on my rings while I slept, and I'd my suspicions about who that was. Who is your top guess?

CHAPTER 16

Mixed News

Good news of the second tumour shrinkage came about December 15, 2008, when Mike's oncologist said, 'Be sure to really enjoy this Christmas.' We'd bought some time. Mike told our boys about the shrinking. Our youngest said, 'Does this mean you will still be around?' Wondering if he would get mad, we braced ourselves. Luckily for all, he laughed, so we all did. We absolutely were all grateful for that Christmas. We never said he was dying, and yet, both kids knew. Kids know and they feel everything that is going on, whether it is around death or something else significant in their life.

I will always remember how sad Mike looked sitting beside the Christmas tree. He was grateful but so sad it was the last at the same time. We didn't know what to do. It was awkward for all of us.

On April 20th, we both had dual emotion. So excited for the prospective parents, but afraid Mike might leave that day. That is one time I was really in denial. I believe Mike was waiting to hear the news. He was not speaking at this time, so he didn't express it in words. We did, however, have people visit from the office that day. I should have phoned to check, but I was probably afraid that would send him away. I am not sure what I was thinking. Mike did not get a chance to meet the baby here on Earth, but I am confident he learned the news from Heaven. We'd made it through September when our nephew was born. We were worried about that day, as Mike was very ill also at that time. We both were afraid Mike and our nephew would change places here on Earth. Once we got past that birth, our minds were on the April baby.

We need research to transform this cancer into one that people survive. There are local support groups and a worldwide organization.

Please consider donating. When we discover more successful treatment, we will make greater progress towards a cure.

For more information, go to:

Pancreatic Cancer Canada
https://pancreaticcancercanada.ca/

World Pancreatic Cancer Coalition
https://www.worldpancreaticcancercoalition.org/

National Pancreas Foundation (US)
https://pancreasfoundation.org/

All of them have some excellent information to share.

Many of these situations will vary by country. Be sure to check with the local authorities.

Final Tips

See a doctor early for best outcomes if you suspect something is wrong.

To keep moving, talk, share, and allow everyone the same opportunity, making sure kids feel comfortable to share their thoughts and feelings. Not talking is harder on people. This also applies to job loss.

Patience is something people often do not have after a loss. I recognize this in people all the time. Lineups at the store were the first place I noticed in myself. As I work with people, and my years of grief increase, I am even more aware. The tiniest thing can be annoying. I have thought a lot about lack of patience. I think we do not want to waste any time. We realize and have experienced how precious life is.

When faced with a terminal illness, you really learn to celebrate small victories like this. We celebrated our fourteenth anniversary while Mike was doing treatment. We decided to have a lemonade toast. There was no use having any other drink. We enjoyed what agreed with him and it was the celebration that mattered, not the drink we were toasting with.

One thing that was suggested was to record the appointment with the oncologist, as with shocking news, one often forgets what they said. They talk and suddenly you are off in another place, present in body but not in mind. The cancer center owned recorders you could borrow. Ten years later, appointments would be easy to record on your cell phone. The opportunity to listen to the appointment again was helpful.

All of this occurred just at the beginning of texting. I had a flip cell phone then and did not know how to text. No one explained how to put in a space. So... I sent a few friends some lengthy paragraph messages. I still remember how much a friend laughed. Texting would have been so much easier when at medical appointments and the hospice. Friends tried to get me to text but learning something like that was too hard then.

Mike could be hilarious during treatment, as he'd always been. One time I needed to help him early one morning, getting ready for the cancer center. Both our nine-year-old and Mike owned the same colour and style of long underwear. My son's were quite a bit smaller, but somehow found their way into Mike's drawer. Mike started to put the small ones on. Now those were interesting to get off. His oncologist got a good laugh, and she recommended wearing his own underwear.

About this time, it became apparent we needed a new popcorn popper. We owned an air popper machine for years and suddenly the top busted. Mike decided he needed to make popcorn, and we were so used to the air popper; it was the only option. For some reason this was a period of time that you could not find one easily. After many shopping trips, I finally found one. It was not very user-friendly. It's very low to the counter, and the popcorn shot mostly straight out rather than down into a bowl. One particularly amusing time, the eldest and I arrived home from hockey to find Mike rushing around the kitchen to find enough bowls and an appropriate one to catch this popcorn. It was like smoke was coming out of his ears; he was so frustrated. We looked at each other but knew better than to laugh. Of course, it seemed after that, air poppers were everywhere.

I wanted to mention the toque we found for Mike that hockey season. He wore it with a large point at the top. Everyone called him the Travel Company Gnome. Ha-ha. It was the perfect name. Everyone enjoyed it. Mike was very easy to spot. It was a bright blue, fitting as that was his favourite colour.

Mike loved lottery tickets. He'd not driven in months. One day, I arrived home to find he'd taken my car somewhere. There were no other drivers in the house. He worried I would not return from hockey in time to buy tickets for that night's draw. It surprised him I was such a great detective. Ha-ha. He parked in the garage, I'm sure with no intention of admitting he'd gone somewhere, but not where I did.

I read a really good book about the end of life. You will find it listed on my website hollyroseholland.com. Many people are in denial about the end of life. I was reading this just before Mike died. As much time as we had, I was still surprised and felt unprepared. There are many topics covered in the book, including signs you will get from the body, which may alert you that the end is near.

Making Meals

I asked the kids if they remembered what we used to eat as a family. Things changed so much over the last few years, starting with a special diet, then diagnosis time, and then the cancer. All of these were unique, and this year during the pandemic, eleven years after his death, I finally remembered we made bread in a bread machine before all of this.

Counselling

I recommend counselling for everyone in the family, kids and adults, even if it seems like everything is going well. Counselling both during and after an illness is ideal. We can all use someone in our corner. Find a counsellor who suits everyone. We had an amazing one that we started with before Mike died. She went on to do a different kind of work at Christmas that first year. We were all a little deflated because she was such a good fit for us. I spent a few years looking for another great fit. I finally reconnected with her and we could see her again. That was just what we needed. Later on, we needed another counsellor and found another awesome one. I can't begin to thank either of them enough. There are so many types of counselling available.

Initially, Facebook helped with some people because it was more comfortable behind a screen. How the counselling occurs does not matter. It is important for people to be participating and reaching out when they need help. Online support is also available. Not everyone is comfortable talking face-to-face. Telephone and text support are other delivery methods. They have excellent ways of staying anonymous, which can make all the difference in counselling.

Job loss has the same requirements for counselling, highly recommended.

Conclusion

One way I could get through each day of Mike's illness was that many of another famous person's words played in my head. I would go over them when I took my shower. That was really the only private time. We are supposed to learn something. I kept asking God what we were supposed to learn. I would tell him how hard it was for all of us. In the beginning of the illness, we felt like we were racing the clock to get things done. Later on, we thought we'd done everything we needed to.

Tension had been high in our relationship. Lack of communication on so many levels was the most contributing factor. At times, we were almost like strangers. Illness, lack of answers, and lack of sleep were also major factors. One child was very ill, which was hard because as the mom, I did everything I could to keep him alive, while I was not available enough to others. I would have done the same for them. As I'm writing it, I'm not sure if I ever said that. I guess that's another communication that was missed. I probably assumed they knew. Later I came to learn how much sleep can enable or disable relationships. I think we were on autopilot for most of our marriage. We were older and probably didn't bounce back as easily.

I was still searching for what we were supposed to learn. Despite everything, we took steps to wipe the slate clean with ourselves and others. Mike called most people right after the diagnosis, so most visited while he was in pain, very ill and before he'd a treatment plan. As we'd a rocky marriage leading up to his illness, I finally figured out we needed to fall in love all over again. It wasn't fair to send him off, feeling even slightly unloved.

We'd simply grown apart. We were both tormented by several broken relationships. I wish we'd both received support back then. We needed to unload in confidence. Stress was a major contributing risk factor. That's why there was no family history of pancreatic cancer. It was also a factor in the time it took to diagnose.

I fell back in love with him, because it was the best thing to do for Mike. It was not the best thing for me, because he was harder to lose. I have had an incredible opportunity to keep on living and I so appreciate it. I relied on daytime television shows being available when I moved to Alberta. Phoning was expensive, there was no social media or texting. I felt so alone. I watched daytime television for normalcy, advice, and keeping current. Two women from daytime television were a welcome, positive influence.

Gratitude has played a huge part in my life. I am grateful for the opportunity to help others and because I have lived to see both of my boys to adulthood. I felt a huge weight when they were young, when the winter roads were terrible and we were driving somewhere when we didn't want to let others down, like hockey games.

Life can and will go on. I hope, if you are in a state of being stuck, you will seek professional help. This applies to job loss as well.

Everything here is based on my personal experience. Time, location and your frame of mind in this moment will all have a huge impact. Life is not always kind, but we can make the most of what we have. It is okay to think through and even write down or talk about all the things you would change, if you could. Give it some time, there is no magic formula how much. What is not okay, is staying there.

Prepare to start fresh and look at the world as if you have just arrived. What will people know you for when you leave this world? Now, start planning how you will get there. I will always include fun and laughter in my life. As we are currently immersed in a pandemic, what really matters may be clearer. Like the rest of the world, I have made changes. Some I always understood were good for me but had not taken enough time to implement. Other changes are not popular; however, they work for me. This includes removing anything that is not for my greater good. It is imperative to allocate the time and execute the requirements to create your own destination.

Until We Meet Again...

(RemembranceQuotes.com)

This was added to Mike's Grave

The Following pages consist of
charts to fill in information
I found to be helpful.

I hope you will find them useful.

Holly

FUNERAL

Date, time and location:

Eulogist(s):

Pallbearers and contact information:

FUNERAL

Casket or cremated?

Final resting type? Buried, vault, home?

Final resting place in the world:

FUNERAL

Caterer and contact information:

Music and hymns. Do they need to be approved?

Video and equipment. Is a video allowed?

FUNERAL

Kids welcome?
(I asked people to bring their kids)

Special items to include in the casket -
according to your comfort level.

Set up for the funeral lunch. Remember
a head table for the immediate family.

FUNERAL

Airport pickups / deliveries.
Accept help for this.

Funeral cards
Decide when to distribute

Decide how much to lower the casket if buried.
Not lowering completely can create anxiety.

FUNERAL

Communicate where you will gather after the lunch to keep everyone together. This is not as simple as it sounds.

When is eulogy allowed? During or before service? Find out before advertising. Adjust the service time accordingly.

Newspaper obituaries. Allow the funeral home to do this. Give information to them.

VISION BOARD

List everything from your bucket list.
Add your goals and dreams in words and
pictures. Paper and electronic are both fun to
create. Update as needed, at least once a year.
Keep it where you will see it every day.

PREPARE A WILL

Having a will is necessary for each person.
This makes decisions after your death much easier.
There are a number of options, which may vary by
country. Verify the rules for your place of residence.

TRAVEL

Before you leave the country, check
your medical and travel insurance. If there
is no coverage, stay close to home.

Parental permission is required to travel with
kids in some countries. If a parent has died,
travel with that parent's death certificate.

FOOD

If you have an illness affecting you, will a special diet help?

Add a naturopath, including traditional and natural medicine to your medical team.

Nutritionist:

PHARMACIST

Find a pharmacist you are comfortable with.
They will be able to advise you about interactions.
They are an amazing source of information.

LONG TERM CARE

Would you have a nurse come in?

Is this financially feasible?

Does insurance cover?

HOSPICE

Hospice or Not?

Where will the remaining family live?

CPSIA information can be obtained
at www.ICGtesting.com
Printed in the USA
LVHW020934301220
675237LV00019B/3332

9 781777 288402